A SIMPLE GUIDE TO
WRITING A NURSING CARE PLAN

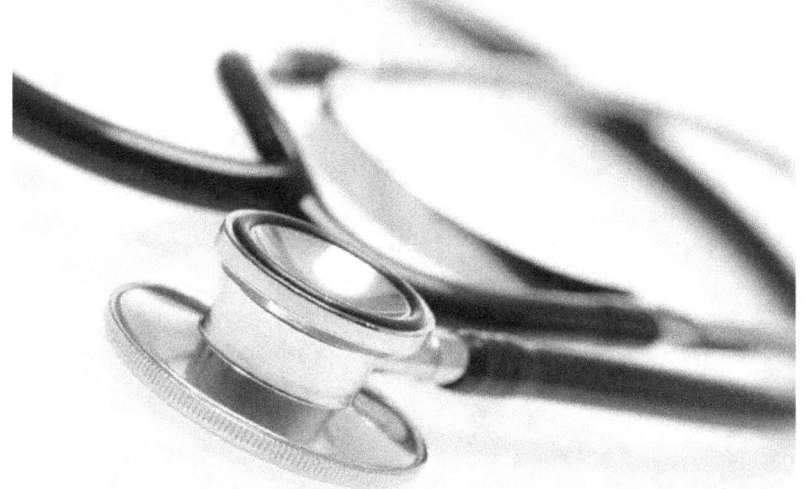

ASHLEY R. HAMPTON
MSN, RN, PCCN

A SIMPLE GUIDE TO WRITING A NURSING CARE PLAN

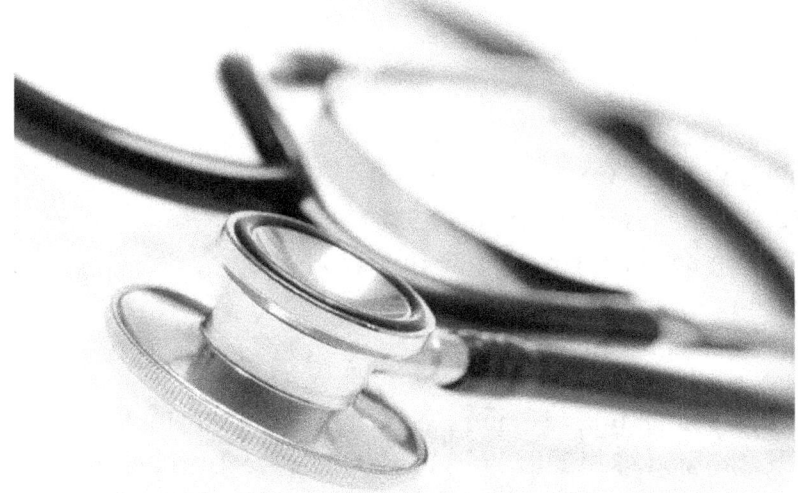

ASHLEY R. HAMPTON
MSN, RN, PCCN

A Simple Guide to Writing a Nursing Care Plan
Copyright © 2017 by Ashley R. Hampton
Electronic Edition: January 2017
Print Edition: March 2017

All rights reserved. No part of this book may be reproduced or transmitted in any form or by any means without written permission of the publisher.

To order products, or for any other correspondence:

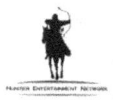

Hunter Entertainment Network
4164 Austin Bluffs Parkway, Suite 214
Colorado Springs, Colorado 80918
Tel. (253) 906-2160 – Fax: (719) 358-9051
E-mail: contact@hunter-entertainment.com
Or reach us on the internet:
www.hunter-ent-net.com

This book and all other Hunter Heart Publishing™, Hunter Heart Kids™ and Eagle's Wings Press™ products are available at Christian bookstores and distributors worldwide.

Chief Editor: Gord Dormer
Book cover design: Phil Coles Independent Design
Layout & logos: Exousia Marketing Group www.exousiamg.com

Print ISBN: 978-1-718653-00-9
eBook ISBN: 978-1-937741-33-4
Printed in the United States of America.

Dedicated & In Memoriam

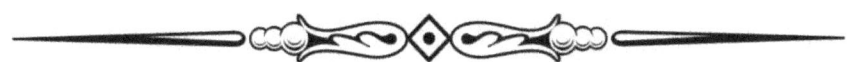

Ella Doris Ricks

and

Virginia Young Summerhill

Table of Contents

Introduction 1
Attention 5
Care Plan Example 7
Reference 11
About the Author 13
Contact & Resources 15

Introduction

A nursing care plan is like a blueprint for providing patient care. My role as a nursing clinical instructor inspired me to produce a universal tool that would simplify the process of developing a nursing care plan. My tool began in the form of an eBook, *A Simple Guide to Writing a Nursing Care Plan*, but expanded in print, as the demand arose for a simplistic, yet detailed approach to writing a nursing care plan.

My book allows the audience to redirect their thinking and focus on what questions to ask when writing a care plan and caring for patients. In return, this will help to improve the quality of patient care. Included is an example of an Acute Pain nursing care plan.

A Simple Guide to Writing a Nursing Care Plan is great for current/future nursing students, nurses, nurse educators, etc. My goal is to reach nursing schools and healthcare facilities nationwide.

A Simple Guide to Writing a Nursing Care Plan

Nursing Diagnosis	Goals	Interventions	Rationales	Implementation	Evaluation
NANDA International, Inc. Approved Nursing Diagnosis (What is going on with the patient? What health concern is your top priority?) **r/t related factors** (What is the pathophysiology of your priority? Avoid the use of a medical diagnosis here.) **AEB** defining characteristics (Characteristics may be subjective or	**ATTENTION:** The type (i.e. long-term, short-term) and number of goals required may vary from institution to institution. Please refer to the note following the tables. What is your expected outcome? What does the patient or family hope to achieve? Goals should be prioritized. Goals should also be	**ATTENTION:** The minimum number of interventions required may vary from institution to institution. Please refer to the note following the tables. What is required of the patient or family to accomplish the goals? What will you do for the patient to help accomplish the goals? How often will these interventions be performed?	**ATTENTION:** The minimum number of rationales and citation format (i.e. APA, MLA) required may vary from institution to institution. Please refer to the note following the tables. There should be a rationale for each intervention. Why are you doing each intervention? How will your interventions help	What did you do for your patient? How did your patient respond to your interventions? What did the patient or family do to help achieve the goals? Refer to your nursing diagnosis, goals, and interventions.	Goal Met, Goal Partially Met, or Goal Not Met? How or Why was the goal met, partially met, or not met? Will you continue, revise, or discontinue the care plan? Re-emphasize your goal. Provide defining characteristics. Be specific!

objective. Be descriptive. How is this particular diagnosis appropriate for the patient? Nursing Diagnosis **r/t** Related Factors **AEB** Defining Characteristics.	measurable, including a time or frequency Be descriptive (Is there a way to assess if the goal was accomplished?)	Like goals, interventions should be prioritized. They should also be measurable, including a time or frequency. Be descriptive. Assess, Do, Teach.	to accomplish your goals? References should be cited.		

Attention

Please follow the nursing care plan policies/guidelines of your employer or institution. This document is not to be substituted for what is required. It is to simply help you understand my thought process of writing a nursing care plan.

If you can understand my thought process, writing a nursing care plan will become easier and faster. Remember to think of your nursing care plan as a blueprint. Be specific! Your care plan should be individualized for each patient. Your nursing diagnosis, goals, and interventions should all be related. Please see my following sample care plan!

Best Wishes,

Ashley R. Hampton, MSN, RN, PCCN

Care Plan Example

Nursing Diagnosis	Goals	Interventions	Rationales	Implementation	Evaluation
Acute Pain r/t traumatic injury of the right humerus and swelling of the nearby soft tissues AEB: Subjective Data- Current Pain 10/10 Tolerable Pain 3/10 Objective Data- Grimacing, Moaning	Short-Term Goal 1. Patient will have a tolerable pain level of 3/10 by the end of the shift. Short-Term Goal 2. Patient will utilize at least 2 non-pharmacologic pain management techniques by the end of the shift.	1-1. Assess pain level every 2 hours and as needed for policy requirements after administering pain medications. 1-2. Administer pain medications every 4 hours per physician's orders and medication administration policy, while also evaluating their effectiveness. 1-3. Educate the patient every 2 hours on reporting	1-1. Assessing pain is the first step in choosing pain management techniques. Pain is what the patient says it is (Gulanick & Myers, 2014). 1-2. Pain medications' side effects and effectiveness should be evaluated individually. Non-opioid analgesics should be given routinely for acute pain. Opioids are used for severe pain (Gulanick & Myers, 2014).	Pain was assessed q2h. In addition, pain was assessed 30 minutes after administration of Morphine 2mg IV and one hour after administration of Percocet 5mg PO, per physician's orders and facility policy. Patient reported relief with pain medications. I educated the patient on reporting pain before it reaches 7/10. Patient verbalized understanding of	1. Goal Met. Continue Plan of Care. Patient reported a pain level of 3/10 by the end of the shift. By the end of the shift, patient was no longer grimacing or moaning. Heartrate-89 BP-126/74 Next available doses of PRN pain medications: Morphine 2mg IV- 8:00pm Percocet

Limited mobility of the right upper extremity

Heartrate -124

BP-170/92 | | pain before it reaches 7/10.

2-1. Assess the patient's willingness to try non-pharmacologic pain management techniques every 4 hours

2-2. Apply cold compress to right upper extremity and provide repositioning support every 4 hours.

2-3. Educate the patient every 4 hours on other forms of non-pharmacologic pain management techniques | 1-3. In an effort to increase pain relief, it is important for patients to report pain early (Gulanick & Myers, 2014).

2-1. Patients may have misconceptions and fears about non-pharmacological pain management techniques (Gulanick & Myers, 2014).

2-2. Cold compresses help to decrease swelling and pain. Repositioning promotes comfort and helps to maintain good body alignment (Gulanick & Myers, 2014). | reporting pain in a timely manner.

I assessed the patient's current knowledge about non-pharmacological pain management techniques.

The patient reported using distraction and guided imagery in the past. In between medication administration, I applied an ice pack to the right upper extremity and helped the patient to reposition. Two pillows were used to support the patients affected extremity.

The patient verbalized that she was comfortable. | 5mg PO-12:00am

2. Goal Met.

Continue Plan of Care.

Patient utilized a cold compress and repositioning, which are both non-pharmacological pain management techniques.

Pain level- 3/10 by the end of the shift. |

				2-3. Patients should be informed that there are multiple pain management techniques (Gulanick & Myers, 2014).	I provided the patient with patient education on non-pharmaco-logical pain management techniques. By the end of the shift, the patient was able to verbalize at least four forms of non-pharmaco-logical techniques.	

Reference

Gulanick, M. and Myers, J. L. (2014). *Nursing Care Plans: Diagnoses, Interventions, and Outcomes.* (8th ed). Philadelphia: Elsevier/Mosby.

NANDA International, LLC. (2017). *Defining the Knowledge of Nursing.* www.nanda.org.

About the Author

Ashley Hampton is from Tuscumbia, Alabama, currently residing in Melbourne, Florida. Ashley juggles three jobs as a Clinical Nursing Instructor, Per Diem Nurse Educator for injection training, and is a staff nurse on a Trauma/Surgical Progressive Care Unit. She also has nursing experience in the Emergency Department, Long-Term Care, and Hospice. Ashley is the wife of her husband, Charles, and also a mommy to her three-year-old son, Xyan. She received both a Bachelor of Science in Nursing (2009) and a Master of Science in Nursing (2015) from the University of North Alabama. She is now enrolled in Kaplan University's Post-Master's Family Nurse Practitioner Certificate Program. Ashley loves her profession.

"Needless to say, I've had my share of nursing care plans!"

~Ashley R. Hampton, MSN, RN, PCCN

Contact & Resources

Ashley R. Hampton, MSN, RN, PCCN
Email:anricks09@gmail.com

Book available in print and eBook format on all major digital outlets, including our website at www.hunter-ent-net.com.

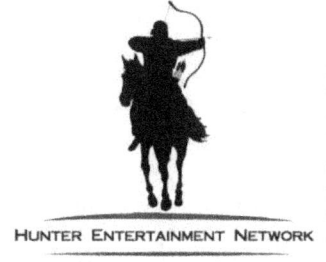

HUNTER ENTERTAINMENT NETWORK

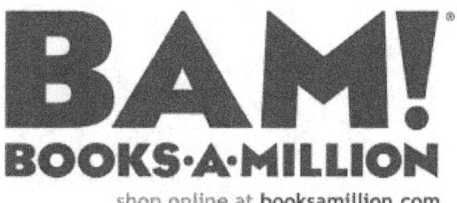

kindle STORE

BARNES & NOBLE
BOOKSELLERS
www.bn.com

www.ingramcontent.com/pod-product-compliance
Lightning Source LLC
Chambersburg PA
CBHW030047230526
45472CB00005B/1710